# WHAT
## IS MY MOTHER
# DOING TO ME?

**A TEENAGER'S JOURNEY TO RECOVERED HEALTH
THROUGH BIOMEDICAL INTERVENTIONS**

**Andrew Luke Zimmerman**

LIBRARY OF CONGRESS CONTROL NUMBER: 2010907488

ISBN: 1452883742

Printed in the United State of America by CreateSpace

Bulk purchases, please contact debbiez@hawaii.rr.com

# What is My Mother Doing to Me?

## Dedication

If I'm going to dedicate this book to someone, I really don't see any alternative but to dedicate it to my mom. After all, this book is the story of what she did for me.

## Disclaimer

I am not a doctor...............just a teenager telling his journey with biomedical interventions. This book should not be interpreted as medical advice. Nor is it a comprehensive guide to biomedical interventions.

Some names, ideas, and facts have been (sort of, not too much) altered to protect me from angry mobs. As awesome as my Mixed Martial Arts (MMA) skill is, I could probably only take one attacker at a time. Also, more names, ideas, and facts were changed for the sake of somewhat-poorly-done humor. More still were changed to write a really confusing disclaimer.

(This page intentionally left blank)

# Acknowledgements

I've always been real confused on the "acknowledgements" page. I've had a couple of problems with it. For one, many authors include a bunch of names that:

A) No one will really care about.
B) No one will read.
C) Will accomplish nothing.

For example, if I listed off a long group of names, and you weren't listed, would you care? Would you bother reading it? Would it accomplish anything? The answer to all those questions is probably "no."

However, at this time of writing, Robert Downey Jr. won a Golden Globe for his performance in "Sherlock Holmes," and during his acceptance speech he said he had "nobody to thank." I do not wish to be such a loser. So, at the risk of boring the reader to death, I decided to write out this page.

First and foremost, I want to thank the Man upstairs. For those of you who don't know, I'm referring to God. I've always known that following religion is good. (With the possible exception of radical Islam, because some followers of radical Islam tend to crash planes, cars, and bombs into giant buildings, killing many people, including themselves, in the process.)

Next, I'd like to thank my mom for all these experiments and what not. I realize I probably despised her to the fullest extent possible, perhaps to the point where I was considering homicide while undergoing biomedical interventions. However, when I look back I see how blessed I am. I would also like to thank her for helping me write this book. (Before you ask, I promise you, she didn't make me write that, as hard as that sounds to imagine.) I would also like to thank her for pulling me out of the public school system to homeschool me. It would have been nice if she did BEFORE I spent about 150 days with about 65-70 kids who hated me.

Next, I would like to acknowledge all the doctors who somehow made me better. I believe that you guys should totally take the rest of the day off. If you want, go ahead and grab a beer. I don't know exactly where you live, so I can't pay for it. And if I did know where you lived, I'd still be underage. So all I can really offer is thanks, and sorry the health care system sucks.

I would like to thank my dad as well. I would say my pop is one of the most awesome people in the world, easily the most influential person I know. If I ever have a problem, generally I go to him, then to my youth pastor, then my mom, then myself, and then I resolve the problem by choosing a Gatorade over a Dr. Pepper.

I know I mentioned this earlier, but I want to give a second thanks to Dr. Jerry Kartzinel. Even though he prescribed me MB12 shots, challenging my last shreds of dignity, he still is the doctor that helped me become who I am today. In this book I often refer to him as "the crazy scientist," but really I know that he is only crazy about helping kids.

The last group of people I would like to thank is the small group of people that lifted me up and prevented my suicide during the 5th grade. These individuals gave me reason to continue living. Though most of them I do not see anymore, should they be wandering around Amazon trying to buy one of those self-help books, and they happen to see my book, I would like to say "thanks." Now buy the book already.

I wrote out a lot more acknowledgements then I thought I would, considering I said I didn't understand them at all. Rather then put more in this text, I'm going to shut up and start the book already.

# Part One: Introduction

# Chapter I

# Welcome to My World.
### *(Does that sound a bit too similar to The Matrix?*
### *Because it's NOT the world of Red Bull)*

My name is Andrew Zimmerman. If you didn't know that, perhaps you should check the cover...actually, not knowing the author's name may mean you can't read. If you can't read, I have no idea why you have this book in your hands. True, there are some pictures later down the line...but they are a tad violent.

For now, I'll try to put my incredibly stupid humor aside and give you an introduction. Before I go over WHO I AM, I'll go over WHO I AM NOT.

a)  A corporation trying to suck in money.
b)  A crazy scientist...........aka DAN! doctor.
c)  A mom who pleads with her kids to follow the ideas sent from a crazy scientist, who might be taking orders from the greedy corporation.
d)  A dad who has to go along with his wife to get his kids to follow stuff sent by the crazy scientist (under the threat of sleeping on the couch).
e)  A kid who has surrendered to his dad's commands, which were sent by his wife, which were sent by a crazy scientist, which were sent by the greedy corporation.

Now, I get to go over WHO I AM.

a)  I'm a 14 year old guy.
b)  I like wrestling.

c) I love fighting in general. Mixed Martial Arts is one of the most awesome inventions of man. I hope to be a professional cage fighter one day.

d) I like staying in shape. (If you have a weight problem, I actually have a weight loss/health optimization in the bonus section of this book.)

e) I like running; my favorite distance is the mile.

f) Sometimes I'll go swimming. It's ok, but mighty boring at times.

g) I like video games. (Guilty pleasure. We all have our problems now, don't we?) My favorite game is Oblivion, because there's basically endless content, and at this writing I'm anticipating the release of Star Wars: The Old Republic.

h) I love metal. You know – the music kind of metal. I recently got an Epiphone. (That's an electric guitar - picture on back cover.) I like Linkin Park, Papa Roach, Evanescence, Ensiferum, Ozzy Osborne, AC/DC, Wintersun, P. O. D, Nitro (Michael Angelo Batio, that's why) and also some rock bands, but only REAL rock bands. By "rock" I do not refer to the Beatles, Genesis, and Chicago. These bands I despise to the maximum. (Please refrain from asking "Does he really hate them, or is he trying to make another real stupid joke?" The answer is, "Yes, I really do hate these bands.") I very much like The Who, Van Halen, and Led Zeppelin, and perhaps Green Day. While a little light, they are quite good.

i) Currently, I'm homeschooled and I love it!

j) I live in Hawaii, but I'm tired of it. I'm tired of how everyone accentuates the culture. There are no theme parks here except one water park (water parks are inferior to roller coasters), and no one ever shuts up about how wonderful

Obama is. I also hate the fact I don't get to see my relatives often. (My mom is from Pennsylvania, and my dad's from Texas. Amazing my family ended in Hawaii, isn't it?) Unlike many people, I have really great relatives I wish I got to see. Hawaii is very isolated. No one really takes that into account whenever they say "Oh, I'd like to move to Hawaii".

k) I'm subject to biomedical experiments and what not.

That should give you a quick rundown on who I am today. Basically, I'm just a normal teenager. Now for my story..............

# Chapter II

# I SAID I WANTED FRIES, NOT EXERCISE.

Throughout my life, I had always been quite low on energy. Even when I was younger, I never had any problems with hyperactivity even when I had eaten every piece of Halloween candy. I also had trouble focusing and paying attention. Finally, I had problems with acid reflux (heartburn). If you have ever experienced heartburn, you know that you actually begin to believe your heart has self-ignited. It is a painful experience.

These problems grew, grew, grew, and grew. I believed they would just keep growing. No end was in sight, but at the time, I really didn't care. Then when I hit 5th grade my problems climaxed.

But let me backtrack. I went to public school in 2nd and 3rd grade and had a wonderful time. Then I decided to switch to a more challenging private school in 4th grade. That was fine, but I missed my old friends, so I went back to public school in 5th grade. That was a huge mistake.

I don't know what happened during the year I went away, but when I returned to public school I felt like most of the kids hated me. I'm not exactly sure as to why, but here is what I had going against me: I couldn't focus, I was a pathetic runner - I gassed out in the exercises very quickly, I was lucky to bench 15-20 lbs, and was the true definition of a wimp. I despised recess and prayed that there would be rain so I wouldn't have to go outside. I loved indoor recess. I would read a book, play a board game, play chess, just about anything to not have to go outside. I hardly had any friends, so it didn't really matter. I'd just play with about anyone who would hop up to the board. Then the guy who ran the indoor recess died. I went through some serious depression. Between hating the outside, not having any friends, an inability to focus, a completely broken school system, and apathetic teachers, I actually considered suicide. Simply put, I had nothing to live for.

One night, I took a kitchen knife and (God, I'm getting a little teary-eyed writing this) went to my room. My whole life had been flashing before me, all I had done…and I tried. It was like my triceps autonomously decided to stop working. I just gave it some more thought. Perhaps I wasn't alone.

I wasn't.

# Chapter III

# All in the Family

**(Lucky me, I don't have an Octomom).**

I come from a family of 4. There's my mom (the one who was extremely pliable to the crazy scientist), my dad (who is very perplexed by biomedical interventions, despite denying it to the ends of the earth - but he's awesome), and my brother, David Zimmerman. (Actually, do you count the guinea pig, Chompers? If so, that would make 5 family members.)

I have an extremely difficult time believing that David and I are actually biological siblings. I have brown hair, he has blonde hair. He loves soccer; I'd rather be water boarded than play that game. I'm a fan of MMA; he'd use boxing in street fights. Also, completely opposite to me, he had *too much energy*, whereas I had *waaay too little*. I would have gladly traded problems with him, but you don't exactly get to pick n' choose. He couldn't sit still and was extremely aggressive. (He even punched teachers for touching him.) Most of the time, he was under the table at school.

My mom quit her job because of the challenges we had, and she took us to a guy I'll refer to as Dr. Jekyll. (I named him Dr. Jekyll because he has no idea of the danger in the pills he prescribes.) I remember talking to him; he seemed to want to understand my mind. However, at the time, I was simply incurable by talk therapy. I remember now when he said "Andrew, you're a kid. Kids have a lot of energy. It's ok to spend energy." The fact was I didn't have any energy, so all Dr. Jekyll was doing was making himself look like a complete idiot. Then Dr. Jekyll comes up and prescribes some sort of stimulant medication (I've never been one to memorize all those fancy names), and sends me on my way. I take it, and suddenly, I can focus. I love the day! The teacher is quite shocked on how I'm doing. I'm a little tired, but I can focus. Recess comes, and because I feel so good about school, I think "Hey, maybe I can run faster as well!" I saw a race that was going on, and I jumped in.

I didn't even make it 40 feet. I collapsed.

I got up slowly and dragged my feet back to the bathroom, and decided to just wait there. Since it was P. E. day, I would be in huge trouble. I saw a jump rope, and when no one was looking, I started beating one particular area of my leg. I remember feeling so much pain, but I knew it would be inferior to the pain I would feel if I participated in PE. Then, with my last strength, I ran over to a tree and smashed my leg into it, creating quite a gash. This was extremely painful. I then proceeded to lie to my teacher about how I was playing tag with some of the younger kids, and I tried to climb a tree and "accidently" scraped my leg. Promptly, I was sent to the nurse, who proceeded to give me a pass out of P. E. I couldn't use the same lie twice though, and dreaded next week.

Anyway, on stimulant medication I couldn't sleep or eat lunch. So, while stimulants worked for my focus, the side effects were intolerable. It was not a workable solution for me. Then a crisis hit.

David, my little brother, got arrested in the 2nd grade while playing dodgeball at recess. He had an incident with a girl whose mom worked for a big law firm. Honestly, I don't think it was that bad. Kids get into squabbles at school all the time. Personally, I believe that the girl's mom had a problem with David, and used this situation to get him in trouble. She called the police and demanded that charges be pressed. David was charged with "harassment." My parents could have made a charge against the girl for 2nd degree "assault," but decided not to because, as they predicted, the trial didn't even get heard. The incident, coupled with my problems, caused my mom to fire Dr. Jekyll (giving me an opportunity to flick him off). We then headed off to California - my mom, my brother, and me. We went to do some kind of brain SPECT scan because there was obviously something wrong.

The brain scans found that the stimulant medication David and I used was THE WORST POSSIBLE medication we could have tried. Stimulants activate the frontal lobe of the brain and our frontal lobes were already highly active. However, there were parts of our brains that had way too little activity.

One of the more interesting outcomes of the brain scan appointment came from a conversation my mom had with another parent in the waiting room. Little did I know this conversation would change my entire life, possibly forever. This parent introduced my mom to DAN! (Defeat Autism Now!). Many kids with special brains ("special" is an extremely nice way of saying "broken") like me, could be helped from biomedical interventions, meaning, quite literally, altering the biochemistry of my body. Because of this, my mom met a DAN!

trained physician, who I will refer to as the crazy scientist, named Dr. Jerry Kartzinel, MD. This is where my journey began in January 2007. I had just turned 11.

# Chapter IV

## I've been told that if I don't make things happen, things will happen to me. I responded by punching this person about the head. *(Robert Collier)*

By this completely unnecessary quote, I mean if I don't try to take control of my life, I can't really control anything, can I? We can't control much of how our lives go, to be quite honest. We can't control past mistakes. We can't control the weather. We can't control the economy (but to help it, buy 60 copies of my book). We can't control the way people act towards us. We can't control the lotto (but that would be truly awesome). But there is one thing we can control. One hope we can hold on to. One thing that separates us from animals. This is our *choice*. We can choose how we will react. Quite honestly, I am so sick and tired of people going off on how we don't have free will. I decided a while back, when someone says "We don't have free will," I would respond by punching them in the head and saying "Ok, then."

The reason I *chose* to go off on that long philosophical rant was not because I was bored, wanted to repel my brother sitting on the desk during this writing, or perhaps look busy when my mom was coming by. I went over that because when my journey began in 2007, I chose to learn whatever I could about why this had happened, and how I should respond to it. I couldn't exactly understand why I was put on a gluten and casein free diet (the story changed every time I'd ask) but I chose to study for an answer. I also elected to investigate why I took more pills than an average senior citizen.............and all the other mysteries surrounding the biomedical movement – which I will attempt to explain in this book.

I've never been diagnosed with autism, nor do I think I was ever autistic.  However, as we got into the biomedical movement I discovered I had some of the same challenges autistic kids have including issues with: digestion, allergies, immune system response, hormones and methylation.  David had the same issues (except for hormone challenges) plus a minor detoxification problem.

So, why didn't my mom explain biomed to me?

For starters, my mom might not have told me very much about biomedical interventions (or changed the subject when I asked) because I was too young to understand.  She hid a lot of problems I never knew I had.  To discover I had A.D.D, I had to look at her report to the crazy scientist, Dr. Kartzinel.  To be perfectly honest with you, I still have not forgiven her for this.  I also haven't forgiven her for lying to me about Santa Claus and for accidentally hitting me with a tennis ball about 2 SECONDS after she promised she wouldn't. (I'm quite a grudge holder.  Is this a bad thing?)

The second reason my mom didn't explain biomedical interventions to me is because she didn't know how to do it.  This is why the story changed every time I asked, but I imagine it's a hard topic to fully understand.

Deep down I knew I had a fantastic brain.  Throughout my life my teachers always told my parents I was "very bright." I could read before I was potty trained. (Actually, I can't remember if I could actually read or not. I might have simply memorized **Cat in the Hat**, tricky me). I could type (well) by around 6, and I did tons of math in my head. Yet I still had problems with focus. It seemed extremely illogical. Then I discovered a conspiracy - a conspiracy that had been hidden from me since birth.

Dr. Martha Herbert, a professor of neurology in Harvard, came up with the idea that autism was a problem with the body that affected the brain. While I didn't have autism, perhaps I had a sick body which prevented my brain from functioning optimally. Perhaps my underlying medical issues were like a conspiracy trapping me in my own little world.

Before I go over my journey with biomed, I want to repeat my disclaimer: I am not a doctor and this is not medical advice. Moreover, no two bodies are alike. What worked for me, may not work for you. What works for you, may not work for me. Partnering with a DAN! doctor, you may try some interventions I didn't. However, there may be some overlap in our journeys.

# Part Two: My Journey to Freedom
*(This felt longer than the Crusades.)*

# Chapter V

# In the Beginning........

One morning, I went to breakfast. My mom wasn't up, so I hopped over to the fridge. It was the day after Christmas. I loved eggnog, so I took out some and poured it into a glass, and let the heavenly taste surround my taste buds. I saw my mom come over and she waited until I finished the glass. As soon as I was done, she took another glass, emptied all the eggnog into it, and drank everything. I had no idea why as my mom never liked eggnog. At first I thought she was simply being mean. I asked her "Mom, you know I love eggnog so much. Why did you drink everything and not share?" From here, the painful reality began. She explained I wouldn't be having it anymore, or any dairy products either. I simply could not understand. I soon realized she had removed all milk from our family diet, and I saw some "Almond Milk" on the counter. I had heard of this "Almond Milk" before, but I thought it was only for lactose intolerants or complete retards. Not me.

David was delivered the same news, and went apes*!?@. David loved milk, and quite literally, drank it more then he drank water. I remember he grabbed the fridge's door, and almost ripped off the handle looking for his precious milk. Not pleased, he grabbed the freezer door, tried the same thing, and found no milk. He slammed both doors closed, shoved me out of the way, and sprinted to the 2nd fridge located in a back closet. There he found his sacred milk, and literally began consuming it out of the carton. I knocked it out of his hand, begged him to try to control himself, and trapped him in a rear bear hug, since at that time I didn't know much about chokes to put him to sleep. Then I simply waited until he stopped attempting to punch me about the head. The night before, we had been on very good terms, (our "terms" are constantly changing, friends one day, wishing for the others death the next), so I had no desire to fight back, but I wanted to do something. Unable to do much, I grabbed his wrist, pulled him out of the back closet, and pinned him against a wall. I'm fairly certain this move permanently altered his psychology, because whenever we are physically fighting now, one of his favorite moves is to grab both wrists, pin one arm against the wall, and drop body shots like crazy.

David's behavior continued to decline for several weeks upon the loss of milk from his diet. How could removing milk from a person's diet cause such an extremely negative behavioral response? It was strange. Eventually though, he calmed down and began showing real improvement. He wasn't getting in many fights at home or school. He wasn't cussing. He was more relaxed, happier, and had better self control. His initial regression upon the loss of milk was similar to watching a heroine addict come off of heroine. But once he lost his urge for casein, he was much better off.

As for me, I didn't mind losing milk so much, but I hated the thought of being denied a staple of the food pyramid. The principle, not the product, sent me into a stage of rage and confusion. Gradually, I got use to the Almond milk, and I couldn't tell the difference between the new "dairy free" butter and old "real butter" so that wasn't much of a problem. In fact, I can't believe that Earth Balance Spread is not butter!

Just as we had adjusted to casein free living, my mom announced wheat was now out of the picture. I thought she was simply making another short term experiment. Perhaps she had just run out of wheat. I was sure it would be over in a week or two.

That was 3 years ago.

I remember a period when I almost worshipped Wheat Thins. I'd have them just about every flippin' day, sometimes just a couple handfuls, sometimes the whole bag. I also loved pizza, and regularly ate Ramen and Mac 'n' cheese. I despised my mom to the fullest extent for a month after losing my gluten. For the last 3 years, I have heard "It's going to be over soon...don't worry..." Now I hear "When you move out, you can make your own decisions."

Forgiving my mom for altering my diet was certainly easier when some good substitutes came in for wheat and dairy. Gradually we found some gluten free/casein free (gf/cf) bread, cookies and cereal that were good. Pamela's gluten free brownies are actually better than Dunkin Hines. Homeschooling definitely made diet compliance easier because the public school system served pizza, chips, and all sorts of illegal stuff. However, if I went back to public school today, I know I could maintain the gf/cf diet by bringing lunch from home.

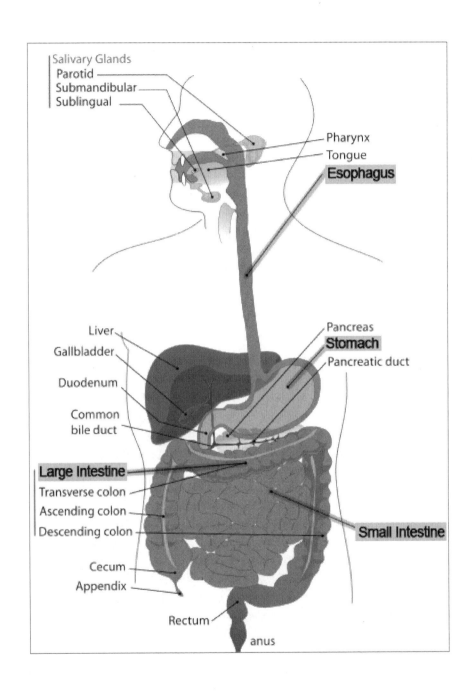

Salivary Glands
Parotid
Submandibular
Sublingual

Pharynx
Tongue
**Esophagus**

Liver
Gallbladder
Duodenum
Common
bile duct

Pancreas
**Stomach**
Pancreatic duct

**Large Intestine**
Transverse colon
Ascending colon
Descending colon

**Small Intestine**

Cecum
Appendix

Rectum
anus

# Chapter VI

# Overview of the Diet

There is no point in telling you something is bad for your digestion if you don't know how the digestive system works. (Please refer to diagram on page 28 while reading this section.) So, here is my explanation............The process begins when you think of something to eat or drink. For the sake of an example, I'm going to say spare ribs. (If you hate spare ribs, you can insert your favorite entrée.) But anyway, you are thinking of spare ribs, the incredible overwhelming awesomeness of its taste in the full... awesomeness (nothing like using the same adjective twice in one sentence to drive a point home) causes you to salivate. (Please do not ask me why this happens when you see a hot guy/girl, because I have no clue. Nor do I want a clue.) Back on topic though, the saliva makes it easier for the food to be digested. Food has to be extremely small throughout this process. Your teeth slice up the meat, and the saliva breaks it down as well. Eventually, you swallow it. It will travel down a small pipe called your esophagus. Because it is narrow, it is the reason you feel like you are going to die whenever you eat something without chewing it well, because you are shoving it down the esophagus. The esophagus crushes the food as it descends, but briefly afterwards, the food hits the stomach for about 20 minutes. Your stomach crushes the food quite well, and after it's had its fun playing trash compactor, the food goes into your small intestine.

I've always been very confused as to why it's called "Small Intestine" because it's about 10-20 feet in length - around 4 times longer then the "Large Intestine." I've been told the small intestine is called "small" because it is much skinnier then the large intestine. If this is the case, why don't we call it the "skinny intestine" and the "fat intestine?"

But I digressed. Anyway, after the small intestine has its chance to crush the living daylights out of the food (similar to how my dignity was crushed by DAN!), the good nutrients from the food are available to the body. They are absorbed by villi - small hair like structures that contain blood vessels - which line the small intestine. Here is what healthy villi look like:

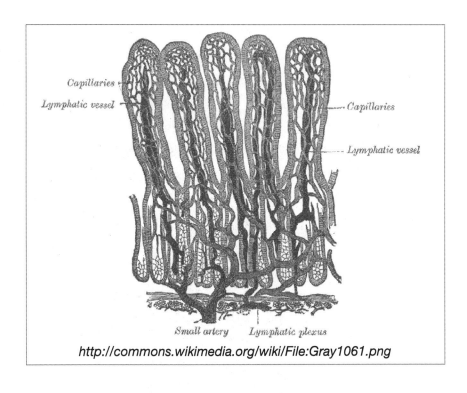

http://commons.wikimedia.org/wiki/File:Gray1061.png

The capillaries in the villi carry nutrients into the blood vessels of the body.

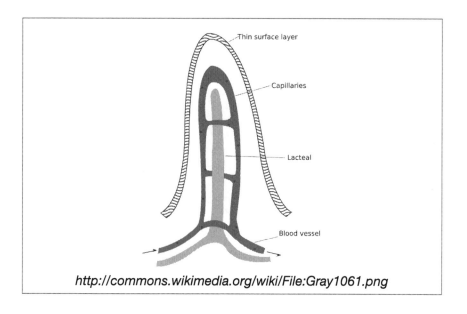

Thin surface layer

Capillaries

Lacteal

Blood vessel

*http://commons.wikimedia.org/wiki/File:Gray1061.png*

The liver then sends it to where it needs to go, giving your body the nutrients it needs. The food/nutrition that is not absorbed by the villi in the small (skinny) intestine proceeds to your large (fat) intestine. Your large intestine then carries the food to your... well, I'll just call it the last stop. And that's the digestive process. (If you prefer the terms "fat" and "skinny" intestine to "large" and "small" intestine tell your friends. If we're lucky this will be a trend that sweeps the nation.)

So, what goes wrong with digestion that requires some people to be temporarily gluten and casein free? There are doctors who theorize that the villi in a subset of people may be not working properly. In some individuals the villi may be covered in mucous (*Ewww!*) or perhaps damaged. With unhealthy villi the body is unable to absorb the nutrition it needs. (Remember, nutrients are carried around the body through your blood stream, and capillaries in the villa provide the gateway for your nutrition from your small intestine.) Worse still, it is speculated that when the villi aren't functioning properly the lining of the small intestine can get damaged and permeable. This means you get small cracks in the lining of your small intestine. These cracks allow undigested food particles to sneak through your gut lining – a condition referred to as "leaky gut."

Undigested food particles outside the lining of the small intestine are detected by the immune system as "danger." Therefore, your body develops antibodies against these food particles and you develop food allergies. Imagine that, being allergic to food that really shouldn't be harmful..........like gluten and casein.

But why are gluten and casein particularly bad? Gluten and casein have humongous proteins, the biggest in the entire food chain. This makes them harder to digest, and it can potentially make you feel uncomfortable. Moreover, these large proteins can bang away at a weak intestinal wall and damage it, contributing to leaky gut. And seriously, who wants that?

Casein is especially bad because if undigested casein proteins leak out of the small intestine it can potentially work like opium on the brain. That's what claimed my brother's mind. His behavioral problems were directly linked to his milk consumption. Once completely weaned off milk most of the school noticed his positive behavior changes.

I'm sorry if I may sound like I'm rattling off on why milk is so bad for you. If you are getting a little bored, are tempted to check around your room, make sure your mom isn't near, and turn on the Xbox 360, I promise I'll pick up the pace in a minute. The reason I went off on that was because I wanted to inflict a phobia like a fricking spider into you. Leaky Gut is BAD. I hate it. If you have it and do nothing about it, I have 4 words for you:

***"I pity the fool"- Mr. T***

While gluten and casein can easily make the digestive system look worse than Shaun White's hair, other food can also create... problems. And believe me when I say "PROBLEMS ARE BAD. VERY BAD. THAT'S THE PROBLEM WITH LIFE. IT'S FILLED WITH PROBLEMS."

# Chapter VII

# Other Food Allergies

There are 2 kinds of allergies I'd like to discuss: IgE allergies and IgG allergies.

To start off, there are IgE food allergies. People with IgE food allergies are very aware of them. Often people with an IgE allergy can not be within the presence of the food that they are allergic to. Exposure to their food allergen creates an immediate and intolerable response ranging from a rash and wheezing to even death. In severe cases people with IgE food allergies carry an "Epi-Pen" which is a shot used to mitigate a negative response to an allergen.

The second type of food allergy is the IgG food allergy. It's more like being sensitive to certain foods. Often these allergies are developed as a result of a leaky gut. Generally, a negative response to these allergens can take hours or days. With an IgG food allergy you may not suddenly break out in a rash or risk death, but with continued long term exposure it may affect your health.

While an IgG food allergy is not as serious as its cousin, the IgE food allergy, they are plenty challenging. Undetected, IgG food allergies can effect your attention, mood, skin and cognitive function.

People with IgG allergies have probably been regularly consuming the foods to which they are now pronounced "sensitive." Learning you have an IgG food allergy to items you love in your diet is devastating. It's hard to eliminate these foods after years of consumption. Often the foods we are most sensitive to are the foods we crave the most. Regardless, IgG food allergies are important to find. So, even if you don't have a history, get allergy tested. You'll thank yourself when you start feeling better. Moreover, often after several months of avoidance, IgG food allergies clear and you can resume eating your old favorites.

# Chapter VIII

# Laboratory Testing

There are thousands of reasons why someone's brain isn't working right. It may be they are a 30 year boxer. It may be because they eat food their brain doesn't respond well to. It may be because they do drugs. Or, it may be other toxin exposure – not a laughing matter. In any case, whatever is keeping your brain from operating in a state of enlightenment can often be determined by laboratory testing. This means you must provide samples of your pee, poop, hair and/or blood so scientists can tell what problems you might have.

Let me get one thing out of the way. LAB TESTING SUCKS. You always feel like a guinea pig. While I admit that it really helped fuel my suicidal thoughts, once I got over my belief I was being used as a Gen-Next pediatrics experiment, I felt significantly better.

This part is going to be very hard for you more sensitive guys and gals. Are you ready? Occasionally blood draws are required. I know some of you are scared of needles, so I'm going to give you some advice. You may want to share this passage with your parents. If you have a fear of needles THIS IS REASONABLE. I have a friend with whom I do MMA. The guy is amazing. He is a good grappler, a fantastic striker, and has a pretty good gas tank. But when he went for a blood draw, he got so scared; he yelled at the nurse who was going to do the draw and threatened to punch her if she stuck the needle in his arm. After he became violent some security guards grabbed him and held him down firmly. Needless to say, the draw never happened.

Back to my original point, your fear is reasonable. Your parents should respect that. This does not give you a complete get-out-of-draw-free pass. However, your parents should accommodate you. On the days that I had blood drawn for laboratory tests, my mom allowed me to spend a little time on my Xbox after the lab visit. You could also ask your parents for a topical anesthetic. A topical anesthetic is a cream that is gently rubbed on the skin where the injection will take place. Its role is to reduce or eliminate any pain associated with the shot. I didn't use one, but I hear they are very helpful for people who are particularly fearful of any type of pain.

Often blood labs are drawn first thing in the morning, before breakfast. This is helpful because usually I was only half awake. When the lab technician (aka blood drawer) called me to her work station, I'd always ask her to wait a moment. Then, I'd use Tai Chi techniques to clear my mind. After about 10 seconds, I'd exhale and say "go." Then, as I inhaled the needle would be inserted. I usually didn't watch this part or it would gross me out.

The poke is the worst part of a lab draw and it only lasts a second. Once the needle is in, a good lab technician will try to initiate conversation to make the short waiting period pass even more quickly. If I got a bland lab technician I'd try to initiate conversation. My favorite line was "So, do you like beer? I've heard a lot of good things about it, and want to try it sometime." This was a surefire way to get a response, but some blood drawers (especially recovering

alcoholics), may not appreciate the question.  Who cares, though?
I'm the one that counts in this situation!

Going back to food allergies, IgG food allergies are often determined
by a laboratory blood draw.  Here were my first lab results:

| Alletess Medical Laboratory | COMPREHENSIVE FOOD PANEL | Toll Free | (800) 225-5404 |
| 216 Pleasant Street | IgG ELISA | MA | (781) 871-4426 |
| Rockland, MA 02370 | Run Date: 03/09/2007 | www.foodallergy.com | |

**PATIENT INFORMATION**

ANDREW ZIMMERMAN
DOB:            12/01/1995
Requisition:    701877
Service Date:   03/08/2007

**PROVIDER INFORMATION**

JERROLD  KARTZINEL MD
PONTE VEDRA BEACH, FL 32082
Telephone:       (904) 543-1288
Collection Date:  03/06/2007

| TEST | SCORE | CLASS | | TEST | SCORE | CLASS | |
|------|-------|-------|---|------|-------|-------|---|
| ALMOND | 0.150 | 0 | | LETTUCE | 0.162 | 0 | |
| APPLE | 0.161 | 0 | | LOBSTER | 0.145 | 0 | |
| ASPARAGUS | 0.185 | 0 | | MALT | 0.194 | 0 | |
| AVOCADO | 0.156 | 0 | | MILK (COW'S) | 0.864 | 3 | *** |
| BANANA | 0.165 | 0 | | MUSHROOM | 0.347 | 2 | ** |
| BARLEY | 0.278 | 1 | * | MUSTARD | 0.161 | 0 | |
| BASIL | 0.172 | 0 | | NUTRA SWEET | 0.140 | 0 | |
| BAY LEAF | 0.163 | 0 | | OAT | 0.155 | 0 | |
| BEAN (GREEN) | 0.153 | 0 | | OLIVE (GREEN) | 0.173 | 0 | |
| BEAN (LIMA) | 0.168 | 0 | | ONION | 0.190 | 0 | |
| BEAN (PINTO) | 0.144 | 0 | | ORANGE | 0.175 | 0 | |
| BEEF | 0.146 | 0 | | OREGANO | 0.172 | 0 | |
| BLUEBERRY | 0.190 | 0 | | PEA | 0.171 | 0 | |
| BRAN | 0.163 | 0 | | PEACH | 0.155 | 0 | |
| BROCCOLI | 0.175 | 0 | | PEANUT | 0.405 | 3 | *** |
| CABBAGE | 0.160 | 0 | | PEAR | 0.167 | 0 | |
| CANTALOUPE | 0.163 | 0 | | PEPPER (BLACK) | 0.179 | 0 | |
| CARROT | 0.169 | 0 | | PEPPER (CHILI) | 0.153 | 0 | |
| CASHEW | 0.151 | 0 | | PEPPER (GREEN) | 0.169 | 0 | |
| CAULIFLOWER | 0.171 | 0 | | PINEAPPLE | 0.222 | 1 | * |
| CELERY | 0.178 | 0 | | PORK | 0.128 | 0 | |
| CHEESE (CHEDDAR) | 0.192 | 0 | | POTATO (SWEET) | 0.168 | 0 | |
| CHEESE (COTTAGE) | 0.249 | 1 | * | POTATO (WHITE) | 0.161 | 0 | |
| CHEESE (SWISS) | 0.208 | 1 | * | RICE | 0.139 | 0 | |
| CHICKEN | 0.169 | 0 | | RYE | 0.254 | 1 | * |
| CINNAMON | 0.130 | 0 | | SAFFLOWER | 0.265 | 1 | * |
| CLAM | 0.158 | 0 | | SALMON | 0.165 | 0 | |
| COCOA | 0.168 | 0 | | SCALLOP | 0.151 | 0 | |
| COCONUT | 0.204 | 1 | * | SESAME | 0.374 | 2 | ** |
| CODFISH | 0.163 | 0 | | SHRIMP | 0.157 | 0 | |
| COFFEE | 0.146 | 0 | | SOLE | 0.153 | 0 | |
| COLA | 0.141 | 0 | | SOYBEAN | 0.187 | 0 | |
| CORN | 0.150 | 0 | | SPINACH | 0.159 | 0 | |
| CRAB | 0.208 | 1 | * | SQUASH | 0.144 | 0 | |
| CUCUMBER | 0.160 | 0 | | STRAWBERRY | 0.175 | 0 | |
| DILL | 0.168 | 0 | | SUGAR (CANE) | 0.153 | 0 | |
| EGG WHITE | 0.237 | 1 | * | SUNFLOWER (SEED) | 0.312 | 2 | ** |
| EGG YOLK | 0.177 | 0 | | SWORDFISH | 0.148 | 0 | |
| EGGPLANT | 0.173 | 0 | | TEA (BLACK) | 0.158 | 0 | |
| GARLIC | 0.160 | 0 | | TOMATO | 0.158 | 0 | |
| GINGER | 0.137 | 0 | | TUNA | 0.149 | 0 | |
| GLUTEN | 0.293 | 1 | * | TURKEY | 0.148 | 0 | |
| GRAPE | 0.193 | 0 | | WALNUT (BLACK) | 0.160 | 0 | |
| GRAPEFRUIT | 0.182 | 0 | | WATERMELON | 0.163 | 0 | |
| HADDOCK | 0.152 | 0 | | WHEAT | 0.311 | 2 | ** |
| HONEY | 0.150 | 0 | | YEAST (BAKER'S) | 0.155 | 0 | |
| LAMB | 0.148 | 0 | | YEAST (BREWER'S) | 0.206 | 1 | * |
| LEMON | 0.171 | 0 | | YOGURT | 0.343 | 2 | ** |

From this lab work you can see that gluten and casein were bad voodoo in my body. The lab results were proof positive that my special diet was a good idea, and not some byproduct of my mother's insanity. As my gut got better, gradually my acid reflux got better too! Also, just so you know, the more IgG food allergies a person has, the more likely they have a leaky gut.

# Chapter IX

# Hope for Eating

One of the most important things to know when on this diet is THERE ARE FOODS YOU CAN EAT! As hard as it may be to imagine, there are some foods this diet does not restrict. True, a good number of foods are removed. But that doesn't mean you must now be more careful than a Weight Watcher. Rather, you just need to make sure your eating the right stuff. I like to have a list of foods I CAN EAT in front of me when I approach the refrigerator. This does put a responsibility on your mom, or dad, to keep the kitchen well stocked with "possibilities" at all times.

Most kids are quite picky eaters, and I am no exception. However, I forced myself to try new foods. (WILLPOWER. It's a huge asset to develop.)

You shouldn't have trouble finding substitutes for most foods, but be sure to experiment with foods you have never tried too. I now love nuts. Before I wouldn't touch them. Today, carrots and almond butter are almost like Reese's Pieces to me. This was a huge shift, but you can make it too! Just be determined!

Whole foods like potatoes, papaya, red/green grapes are delicious. Still, one problem remains. Vegetables. I've always hated them, but I can stomach them now. I don't look forward to eating them, but I realize that they get me in with the women, and everything needs sacrifice now, doesn't it?

There is good news, though. The good news is *the diet does not have to be forever*. (If you have celiac disease, however, I'm afraid wheat abstinence will probably be forever for you.) By the time you've finished biomed, however, you probably will have been off your old foods so long you no longer miss them.

# Chapter X

# Supplements

The problem with "Leaky gut" is you don't digest food fully. As a result, supplements are needed to optimize your health and your ability to beat people's head in, or have your own head working properly. They are also good for people who "can't find the time" to eat balanced meals. Over the years, I've gotten accustomed to swallowing every pill in my vitamin cup in one giant swallow. (We're talking a little over a dozen pills here.)

I acknowledge that pills are needed no matter how old you are, but as with everything, your parents must listen to you. My parents did not listen to me, so I plan to get revenge by sending them to a nursing home (Tricky me). Also, if ANY pill for ANY reason gives you ANY bad reaction find out what it is and bring it up to your doctor.

To determine which supplements I should take, my DAN! doctor ordered a Red Blood Cell Elements test. Unfortunately, it too requires a blood draw. Here are my results:

Next Page ⇨

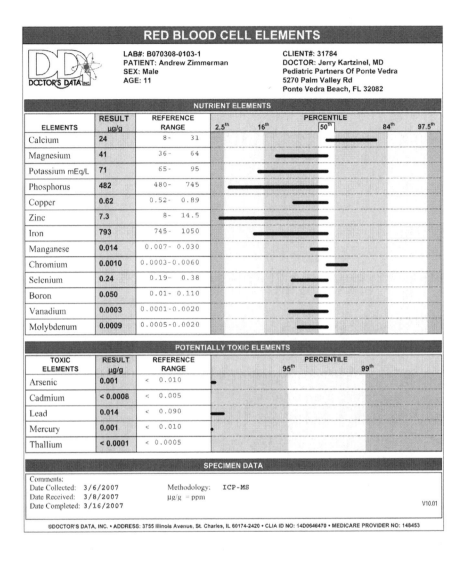

## RED BLOOD CELL ELEMENTS

LAB#: B070308-0103-1
PATIENT: Andrew Zimmerman
SEX: Male
AGE: 11

CLIENT#: 31784
DOCTOR: Jerry Kartzinel, MD
Pediatric Partners Of Ponte Vedra
5270 Palm Valley Rd
Ponte Vedra Beach, FL 32082

### NUTRIENT ELEMENTS

| ELEMENTS | RESULT µg/g | REFERENCE RANGE | PERCENTILE |
|---|---|---|---|
| Calcium | 24 | 8 - 31 | |
| Magnesium | 41 | 36 - 64 | |
| Potassium mEq/L | 71 | 65 - 95 | |
| Phosphorus | 482 | 480 - 745 | |
| Copper | 0.62 | 0.52 - 0.89 | |
| Zinc | 7.3 | 8 - 14.5 | |
| Iron | 793 | 745 - 1050 | |
| Manganese | 0.014 | 0.007 - 0.030 | |
| Chromium | 0.0010 | 0.0003 - 0.0060 | |
| Selenium | 0.24 | 0.19 - 0.38 | |
| Boron | 0.050 | 0.01 - 0.110 | |
| Vanadium | 0.0003 | 0.0001 - 0.0020 | |
| Molybdenum | 0.0009 | 0.0005 - 0.0020 | |

Percentile columns: 2.5th, 16th, 50th, 84th, 97.5th

### POTENTIALLY TOXIC ELEMENTS

| TOXIC ELEMENTS | RESULT µg/g | REFERENCE RANGE | PERCENTILE |
|---|---|---|---|
| Arsenic | 0.001 | < 0.010 | |
| Cadmium | < 0.0008 | < 0.005 | |
| Lead | 0.014 | < 0.090 | |
| Mercury | 0.001 | < 0.010 | |
| Thallium | < 0.0001 | < 0.0005 | |

Percentile columns: 95th, 99th

### SPECIMEN DATA

Comments:
Date Collected: 3/6/2007
Date Received: 3/8/2007
Date Completed: 3/16/2007

Methodology: ICP-MS
µg/g = ppm

V10.01

©DOCTOR'S DATA, INC. • ADDRESS: 3755 Illinois Avenue, St. Charles, IL 60174-2420 • CLIA ID NO: 14D0646470 • MEDICARE PROVIDER NO: 148453

If you look at my lab results, most of my required elements were less then 50%. (To read the chart start at the 50% mark and read the line left or right to see my score.) Sure, my calcium looked great, but take a look at my zinc! It was lower than 2.5%. An addage I've heard a lot is, "If you don't have zinc you can not think."

Here are the supplements I started with. (Mind you, I didn't start every thing at once. Rather, mom added new supplements gradually over time.)

Supplement: Multi Minerals
Benefit: Looking at my Red Blood Cell Elements results you can see that my current nutritional levels were not going to make me a champion! I needed more minerals.

Supplement: Multi Vitamins
Benefit: Keeps you healthy!

Supplement: Calcium/Magnesium
Benefit: Calcium was important because milk was removed from my diet. As a growing boy, I needed a supplement to help build my bones. Magnesium is helpful for many cellular processes, including keeping your mind calm.

Supplement: Zinc
Benefit: Extra zinc was required for me because my lab work showed I was extremely deficient.

Supplement: Fish Oil
Benefit: Did you know that most of your brain is made up of fat? This fat helps keep your brain cells nice and plump and talking to each other. Fish oil really helps with attention.

Supplement: Probiotics
Benefit: Probiotics help fix broken digestion systems, like mine. In short, it crams up your intestine with good bacteria that likes and

supports you (yea!) while it muscles out the bad bacteria causing you harm. (*Yea again!*) Yogurt prides itself on its probiotic content – but most is not casein free.

Supplement: Digestive Enzymes
Benefit: Digestive enzymes also help with leaky gut. These enzymes help to break down food so that your body absorbs more nutrients.

Supplement: Vitamin D
Benefit: Outstanding for immune support.

Note that I had to take several pills for most of the supplements listed above. Often I was taking supplements multiple times per day. Over the years my mom would give me new supplements as suggested by my DAN! doctor. Likewise, sometimes she'd give me supplements she'd read about in books. Occasionally the pills would be a waste of her money. But other times she would hit a winner..............like D-Ribose and L-Carnitine for energy.

If you have trouble swallowing pills, most people will say to put them in your mouth first, and then take a big drink of water. This didn't work for me. What I do is shake up my pill cup so there aren't any pills stuck to the bottom, take a drink of water FIRST (but don't swallow it yet), then pour the pills in my mouth and swallow. The reason I preferred to drink water before inserting the pills is because some of the pills taste awful. With water in my mouth, the pills float around without sticking to my tongue.

If you still have trouble swallowing pills, give your pill the old slice and dice. Some supplements come in a liquid form, but some don't, so you better learn the fine art of pill swallowing. If you can swallow your food at the dinner table, I guarantee you can swallow a pill!

# Chapter XI

# MB12

### *(Methylcobalamin B12)*

When I first started biomedical treatments, there was one intervention that was particularly challenging. In fact, because this treatment was so distasteful I was absolutely positive I could win in a court case against my folks for child abuse. (Yes, I really was thinking about suing my parents. To this day, I still think I could have won.) The area where I believed I had the strongest case was with regard to the administration of MB12 shots. (Basically this is a B12 vitamin delivered with methylcobalamin.) MB12s are shots given by your parents and placed into your arse. Regretfully, this is the best way for the body to absorb the vitamin. However, with this intervention I thought my mom had "crossed the line."

I posted my objection to these shots on the internet and asked what I should do. Some people responded I should report my mom to the police. I considered it. Eventually, I brought my opposition up to her and she seemed very angry I was being this "defiant." We had a huge fight. (Again, take note parents who happen to be reading my book. You'd better make sure that your relationship with your kids isn't shaky because there will be... problems.) While I do believe MB12s work after using them for a while, I ABSOLUTELY INSIST to parents, whatever you do, DO NOT, UNDER ANY CIRCUIMSTANCES, force your child to take MB12s.

Having said all that, as distasteful as it may seem, I do suggest that kids agree to try MB12 shots if their doctor prescribes it. For me they helped tremendously with focus and energy. And with more focus and energy, my interest in socialization increased too! Previously I had been kind of introverted and Dr. Jekyll told my mom that while she was an extravert, she should respect that I was shy. Ha! Once I started feeling better with MB12 we all discovered that I was an outgoing, social guy!

Anyway, if you are prescribed MB12 shots you may need to take it for 2-3 months before this intervention "kicks in." If you don't feel a difference after the trial period, you can always stop. However, if you stop taking MB12 shots and notice a decline in your focus and energy, TAKE IT AGAIN. Period. This is one part you will just need to grin and bear. For me, MB12 was one of the most effective interventions we used.

# Chapter XII

# Hormones

I'm sure you've heard all about hormones in health class (assuming your school has one. If you don't have one, it's a good thing you are reading this book.) Hormones are like chemical messengers that tell your body what to do. They are actually very important for your body to feel well synchronized. The body has over 20 types of hormones, and no hormone can do another's job. (Duh... can a plumber become a cage fighter?)

There are many glands in your body that produce certain hormones, including:

1) Pineal Gland- this gland helps you sleep by producing the hormone melatonin.
2) Adrenal Gland –this is my favorite. It creates the hormone adrenaline. I feel like a god when my adrenaline in flowing.
3) Pancreas – the organ that seemed useless to you when you were in 2nd grade learning about the digestive system. In reality, the hormone insulin is produced in the pancreas and this helps control your blood sugar.
4) Thyroid Gland- this gland helps turn food into energy for you by producing a hormone called thyroxine.

In the area of hormones, I had trouble with my thyroid gland. Prior to the start of biomedical interventions, I spent a lot of time on the couch and lacked passion for life. My Dan! doctor decided to give me a thyroid test. (Yes, another blood draw.) Turns out that was a good idea as the lab results proved my thyroid was not working properly.

The doctor looked at 3 areas: T3, T4, and TSH. I'm not sure what those markers mean, but as evidenced by my skyrocketed TSH number, my thyroid was not working properly. While an ideal number for TSH is around 1.0 - 1.5, I had hit 4.53! (A lower number is better in this case.) Pinpointing the problem is halfway to solving it, which is why labs are so important.

As a result of these labs, I was placed on Armor Thyroid. While I hate to have my life tied to a 1/2 inch pill, it does help my energy and focus A LOT with no side effects. It's amazing Dr. Jekyll put me on stimulant medication when I clearly told him I had energy problems... good thing we got him out of the picture.

FROM: DIAGNOSTIC LAB SERVICES

**DIAGNOSTIC LABORATORY SERVICES, INC.**

650 IWILEI ROAD, SUITE 200
HONOLULU, HI 96817 • TEL PHONE 589-5100

REPRINT

| ADDITIONAL COPY TO |
| --- |
| ZIMMERMAN, ANDREW |
| 3454 SIERRA DR |
| HONOLULU, HI   96816 |

| PATIENT |
| --- |
| ZIMMERMAN, ANDREW |
| DR.: KARTZINEL, JERROLD |

| AGE, DATE OF BIRTH | SEX |
| --- | --- |
| 11, 12/01/1995 | M |

| PATIENT ID | DATE COLL. | REPORT DATE | ACCESSION |
| --- | --- | --- | --- |
|  | 03/06/2007 06:50 | 03/26/2007 05:00PM | YA11422275 PAGE 6 |

| Tests | Results | Reference Values |
| --- | --- | --- |

**Laboratory Notes:**
KARTZINEL, JERROLD M.D. 5270 PALM VALLEY RD PONTE VEDRA FL 32082 ph:9045431288

| | | | |
| --- | --- | --- | --- |
| **Free T3** | 3.3 | pg/mL | 2.5-3.9 |
| **Free T4** | 0.9 | ng/dL | 0.6-1.7 |
| **TSH** | 4.53 | H    uU/mL | 0.28-4.02 |

# Chapter XIII

## To win the Battle of Your Body, You Must: Search and Destroy.

At this point, my mom wanted me to write out some lame analogy relating scary things from the Wizard of Oz into scary things in your body. I had a different idea. I decided I would write an analogy of a ruined iPod. Just like you can put great stuff in an iPod, such as Ozzy Osbourne, Lead Zeppelin, AC/DC, and Linkin Park, you can also ruin an iPod with... bad stuff (I decided not to list names). It is all a matter of what you choose to put inside that little box. If you put in good stuff, you will get to experience its awesomeness. If you put in bad stuff, you will have to wait until you can get back to your computer and put back in the good stuff. The flaw with my analogy is it takes longer then a couple minutes to change from bad to good when working with biomedical interventions. Some of these scary things take years to resolve. They are things like yeast, bacteria, viruses and parasites.

## Yeast

Yeast are parasitic, spore producing devils in your body. Some are fine and found in the body naturally. But my little brother and I had yeast overgrowth, likely several times greater then average.

People respond to yeast overgrowth differently. For me, yeast overgrowth caused attention and focus problems. I remember claiming I was meditating, but my life was basically like a foggy windshield. Also, I craved sugar – as sugar feeds yeast.

David's yeast was bad in every sense of the word. His yeast made him hyper and silly. His stomach was quite bloated, but the rest of his body was very slender. His sensory system was way off balance. He was very sensitive to being lightly touched. (He would punch people for touching him.) Yet, he would hug the living daylights out of unsuspecting victims. Additionally, he was sensitive to sound and would throw a fit if the movie theater was too loud.

Yeast overgrowth can be measured by a Comprehensive Digestive Stool Analysis – a poop test. We started on antifungal medication to kill yeast. It worked *really* well for both of us. Just look at how David's behavior ratings from school improved in only 3 months after he started a gluten/casein free diet and antifungals:

# David's Behavior Evaluation at School

Personal Development

- __2__ Interacts properly with peers
- __2__ Treats others in a courteous manner
- __1__ Works cooperatively with classmates ⬅
- __1__ Is respectful toward adults
- __2__ Shows respect for others' personal space and property
- __2__ Gives others the opportunity to speak in conversations and discussions
- __2__ Tolerates differing perspectives
- __3__ Is open to compromise
- __1__ Shows empathy toward others ⬅
- __1__ Is appropriately assertive
- __2__ Exhibits good sportsmanship
- __3__ Follows through on agreements
- __1__ Exhibits leadership abilities ⬅
- __1__ Demonstrates self-awareness
- __2__ Has an even temperament
- __2__ Handles frustrations well
- __2__ Uses suitable problem-solving strategies
- __1__ Accepts responsibility for behavior and choices
- __2__ Forgives and moves on
- __1__ Apologizes willingly when in error

*David on Stimulants 6/06*

Personal Development

- __3__ Interacts properly with peers
- __3__ Treats others in a courteous manner
- __3__ Works cooperatively with classmates ⬅
- __4__ Is respectful toward adults
- __3__ Shows respect for others' personal space and property
- __3__ Gives others the opportunity to speak in conversations and discussions
- __2__ Tolerates differing perspectives
- __2__ Is open to compromise
- __4__ Shows empathy toward others ⬅
- __2__ Is appropriately assertive
- __2__ Exhibits good sportsmanship
- __3__ Follows through on agreements
- __3__ Exhibits leadership abilities ⬅
- __2__ Demonstrates self-awareness
- __2__ Has an even temperament
- __2__ Handles frustrations well
- __2__ Uses suitable problem-solving strategies
- __2__ Accepts responsibility for behavior and choices
- __2__ Forgives and moves on
- __2__ Apologizes willingly when in error

*David off stimulants 3 months on gf/cf diet and antifungals*

Scale: 1 = Lowest Score/ 4 = Highest Score (Best Score)

Some people initially have a poor reaction to antifungals when the yeast are "dying off." If you do, please note IT'S WORKING. It'll just be bad for a short while before it gets better. You can use Activiated Charcoal 2-3 hours after supplements in the interim.

David and I had to stay on prescription antifungals for almost 2 years before we were able to wean off of them. (We've been off for a year at this writing.) While taking antifungals our doctor regularly checked our liver enzymes to make sure our livers were happy. We never had a negative side effect from this medication which made a lasting improvement in our lives.

## Bacteria

Did you know there are over 500 different kinds of bacteria in your gut? That's right, over 500. Before you attempt sword-swallowing, let me tell you that some bacteria are good. Some bacteria are bad though, and that can wreck you like Tarja Turunen wrecked Nightwish when she got fired. Bacteria can also cause you to have aggression, and the only good time to be aggressive is at a rock/metal concert.

The Comprehensive Stool Analysis can determine the amount of good and harmful bacteria in the gut. To drop a nuke on these bacteria (if you are Japanese, I did not mean to offend you), you'll need an antibiotic. But you have to be careful, because antibiotics wipe out both good and bad bacteria. Moreover, when bacteria die, yeast see the vacant space and move in. So, whenever David and I took an antibiotic, we would also take an antifungal to keep the yeast in check.

# Parasites

Parasites have got to be my most hated (for you over-optimists, I'll call it "least favorite") single celled organisms because they damage me as they feed off me. (Proof that math is wrong- because double negatives here don't produce anything positive. It's the same with grammar.) Generally, parasites give nothing back, similar to *American Idol*.

I was given a stool test to look for parasites. When I found out I had some, I was eager to kill the bloodsucker, despite the pill being disgusting. When the parasites were annihilated I felt much better.

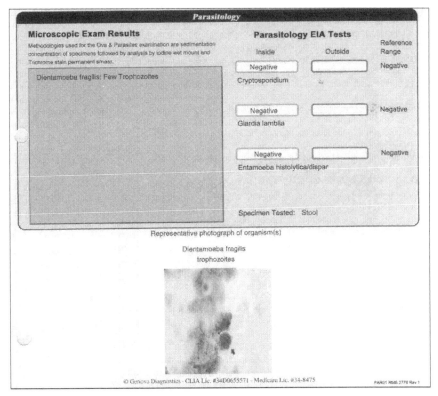

**Parasitology**

**Microscopic Exam Results**

Methodologies used for the Ova & Parasites examination are sedimentation concentration of specimens followed by analysis by iodine wet mount and Trichrome stain permanent smear.

Dientamoeba fragilis: Few Trophozoites

**Parasitology EIA Tests**

| | Inside | Outside | Reference Range |
|---|---|---|---|
| Cryptosporidium | Negative | | Negative |
| Giardia lamblia | Negative | | Negative |
| Entamoeba histolytica/dispar | Negative | | Negative |

Specimen Tested: Stool

Representative photograph of organism(s)

Dientamoeba fragilis
trophozoites

© Genova Diagnostics - CLIA Lic. #34D0655571 - Medicare Lic. #34-8475

PAR01 RMS 2778 Rev 1

Treating parasites can help resolve fatigue, rashes, night sweats, and headaches among other things.

## Viruses

Finally, there are also viruses, but you've surely heard of them. They cause measles, chickenpox, and many other things I chose not to list. They are so small, they can actually infect bacteria. Again, they are nasty little germs that NEED TO DIE. Fortunately, there are also anti-viral drugs and natural supplements to take 'em out.

Viruses attack cells, negatively impact brain function, and basically make you feel crummy. Lab tests can give you a clue whether you have a viral issue; but viruses can be very stealth and difficult to identify.

In summary, your body is a battlefield for good and evil. If you are loaded with the bad stuff – yeast, bacteria, parasites, and viruses - it's not a battle your body can win because your immune system will be extremely overwhelmed. You will need to bring in extra troops for an artillery strike (still working on cool metaphors). Talk to a DAN! doctor who can load your cannon with appropriate medications and supplements.

# Chapter XIV

# The Heaviest Metal Ever

If you have read this book front to back, by now you should have figured out that I like Heavy Metal. When I'm in the gym I'll blast it off and run much more effectively. Heck, I'm even listening to it as I write this book.

I'm in a rock band with some friends, and while I'm sure they disagree with some of my music tastes, they usually go along with the suggested music I bring to practice. I love all types of heavy metal: melodic metal, symphonic, white/black (Yes, sometimes I listen to black metal. If you have a problem with that email me at evilhamster@hawaii.rr.com and we'll fight after school.) I like thrash and speed metal, as well as the old 70s stuff. I like all types of metal............

Except for heavy metal in my body.

Now I'm totally cool with hearing a rock concert inside my head (because there basically is one all the time), but by metal inside my body I mean metals you can touch like tin and lead. I'm also referring to arsenic, mercury, cadmium, thallium, antimony and some other bad metals.

To get a good understanding of what I'm talking about, we need to look at chemistry. (Not the dating game, although there's a time for everything.) In chemistry an "element" is something that can't be broken down any further. Several RPG-loving, chip crunching, fatheads I know would tell you that there are four elements: earth, fire, water, and air. If you see them, please mercilessly beat their dignity and intelligence by explaining that there are 117 elements, not four.

Further, water is not an element. An element is the most simple type of substance. All of the atoms of an element are made of nothing but the element itself. Water is produced when 2 "hydrogen" atoms combine with one "oxygen" atom. Since water can be divided into hydrogen and oxygen - water is not an element. However, hydrogen is an element because hydrogen is made up of nothing except for hydrogen. Likewise, oxygen is an element because it is composed of nothing by oxygen.

Hydrogen, oxygen and all the other elements known to man are listed in the Periodic Table of Elements.

## Periodic Table of the Elements

| 1 | 2 | 3 | 4 | 5 | 6 | 7 | 8 | 9 | 10 | 11 | 12 | 13 | 14 | 15 | 16 | 17 | 18 |
|---|---|---|---|---|---|---|---|---|----|----|----|----|----|----|----|----|----|
| 1 H 1.01 | | | | | | | | | | | | | | | | | 2 He 4.00 |
| 3 Li 6.94 | 4 Be 9.01 | | | | | | | | | | | 5 B 10.81 | 6 C 12.01 | 7 N 14.01 | 8 O 16.00 | 9 F 19.00 | 10 Ne 20.18 |
| 11 Na 22.99 | 12 Mg 24.30 | | | | | | | | | | | 13 Al 26.98 | 14 Si 28.09 | 15 P 30.97 | 16 S 32.07 | 17 Cl 35.45 | 18 Ar 39.95 |
| 19 K 30.10 | 20 Ca 40.08 | 21 Sc 44.96 | 22 Ti 47.88 | 23 V 50.94 | 24 Cr 52.00 | 25 Mn 54.94 | 26 Fe 55.85 | 27 Co 58.93 | 28 Ni 58.69 | 29 Cu 63.55 | 30 Zn 65.39 | 31 Ga 69.72 | 32 Ge 72.61 | 33 As 74.92 | 34 Se 78.96 | 35 Br 79.90 | 36 Kr 83.80 |
| 37 Rb 85.47 | 38 Sr 87.62 | 39 Y 88.91 | 40 Zr 91.22 | 41 Nb 92.91 | 42 Mo 95.94 | 43 Tc (97.91) | 44 Ru 101.07 | 45 Rh 102.91 | 46 Pd 106.42 | 47 Ag 107.87 | 48 Cd 112.41 | 49 In 114.82 | 50 Sn 118.71 | 51 Sb 121.75 | 52 Te 127.60 | 53 I 126.90 | 54 Xe 131.29 |
| 55 Cs 132.91 | 56 Ba 137.33 | 57 La 138.91 | 72 Hf 178.49 | 73 Ta 180.95 | 74 W 183.85 | 75 Re 186.21 | 76 Os 190.23 | 77 Ir 192.22 | 78 Pt 195.08 | 79 Au 196.97 | 80 Hg 200.59 | 81 Tl 204.38 | 82 Pb 207.2 | 83 Bi 208.98 | 84 Po (208.90) | 85 At (209.99) | 86 Rn (222.02) |
| 87 Fr (223.02) | 88 Ra (226.03) | 89 Ac (227.03) | 104 Rf (261.11) | 105 Ha (262.11) | 106 Sg (263.12) | | | | | | | | | | | | |

| 58 Ce 140.12 | 59 Pr 140.91 | 60 Nd 144.24 | 61 Pm (144.91) | 62 Sm 150.36 | 63 Eu 151.97 | 64 Gd 157.25 | 65 Tb 158.93 | 66 Dy 162.50 | 67 Ho 164.93 | 68 Er 167.26 | 69 Tm 168.93 | 70 Yb 173.04 | 71 Lu 174.97 |
|---|---|---|---|---|---|---|---|---|---|---|---|---|---|
| 90 Th 232.04 | 91 Pa 231.04 | 92 U 238.03 | 93 Np (237.05) | 94 Pu (244.06) | 95 Am (243.06) | 96 Cm (247.07) | 97 Bk (247.07) | 98 Cf (251.08) | 99 Es (252.08) | 100 Fm (257.10) | 101 Md (258.10) | 102 No (259.10) | 103 Lr (262.11) |

Some elements are essential for a person to have, in reasonable quantities, to be in good health. These include:

| | | | |
|---|---|---|---|
| • Calcium | • Zinc | • Selenium | • Magnesium |
| • Iron | • Boron | • Potassium | • Manganese |
| • Vanadium | • Copper | • Chromium | • Molybdenom |

NOTICE: All these elements are detected in the Red Blood Cell Elements laboratory test discussed in the "Supplement" section of this book!

Good elements move into your system through the food supply. That's why it is important to eat as much "whole food" (i.e. real food that grows in gardens) as possible.

But just as there are good elements for your body, as I mentioned earlier, there are bad elements too. These elements come in the form of heavy metals and other toxins. Examples of toxic elements include arsenic, cadmium, lead and mercury. They can do radical damage to your body and brain.

How do heavy metals and toxins get inside you? There are many ways:

- Pesticides – Pesticides can be on the food we eat. Pesticides are great for killing bugs, but do you think they are safe for your body? Some people process these toxins just fine, but for others they can create problems. Therefore, it is best to eat organic if you can afford it. But no one has infinite pockets so don't feel bad if you can't.  Just wash your fruits and vegetables well.

- Arsenic in chicken – Many conventional chicken farmers use arsenic in their chicken feed to plump up their animals and make them grow more quickly.  This arsenic can be passed to you upon consumption of chicken that is not organic.

- Environmental pollutants – I don't want to elaborate on this because you will get real bummed out and likely return this book.  I don't want to be like those fear mongering Y2K or 2012 end of the world folks...........but toxins exist in:
  - Air pollution
  - Aluminum cookware or non-stick cookware like Teflon that is peeling.  (If your pan is flakin' you shouldn't be bakin' in it.)
  - Many cleaning products

- Mercury amalgam dental fillings – You know, the gray stuff some dentists still use to fill cavities.  There is no question the gray material contains mercury – one of the most toxic substances on the planet.  Some holistic dentists theorize that this mercury gets released every time you chew!

- Vaccines – Vaccines can be a very controversial source of toxins. It's a well known fact that many childhood vaccines contained mercury (in the form of thimerosal) prior to 2002.  Some forms of vaccines today – like the flu, H1N1 and tetanus shots – still have thimerosal in them. Several normally developing children I know had vaccine reactions that cost them dearly.  Educate yourself by reading books like:

- **What Your Doctor May Not Tell You About Children's Vaccinations** by Stephanie Cave, MD.
- **Evidence of Harm:  Mercury in Vaccines and the Autism Epidemic – A Medical Controversy** by David Kirby.

And if you've ever had a vaccine reaction, seizures, neurological problems, severe allergies or immune system disorders you should do extra homework!

Chelation is one method used to detoxify (remove) heavy metals from the body.  Many kids and families believe that chelation is an important part of recovery for autistic, and occasionally ADHD, kids.  Unfortunately, chelation can deplete your body of essential minerals, so you must be careful to ensure you do this intervention under the guidance of an experienced, licensed doctor.

There are both natural detoxifers and prescription chelators. Natural detoxifers  include Vitamin C, garlic and glutathione.  Others that may need a prescription are ALA, TTFD and OSR.  Prescription chelators include DMSA, DMPS and EDTA.  (I've given you all of the short names for these natural detoxifers and chelators because that's what most people call them.  Only doctors and hyper-vigilant parents know and maybe even care about the long names.)

Natural detoxifers and chelators can be administered in a number of different ways.  Some come as a topical lotion or a pill to be swallowed.  Others come as suppository or IV form.

BOTTOM LINE – Work with your doctor to determine if you have a heavy metal problem and when your body is prepared for chelation. (Generally there is a lot of preparatory work to be done including having a good diet and supplementation in place, plus making sure that yeast, bacteria, parasites, and viruses are under control.)

My brother and I didn't have many problems with heavy metals, but I'm covering this because many people do.  We are all unique..... and that's a good thing too.  If everyone in this world was a copy of me...........there would be no more art, classical music or vegetables!

# URINE TOXIC METALS

LAB#: U080124-0325-1
PATIENT: Andrew Zimmerman
SEX: Male
AGE: 12

CLIENT#: 31784
DOCTOR: Jerry Kartzinel, MD
Pediatric Partners Of Ponte Vedra
5270 Palm Valley Rd
Ponte Vedra Beach, FL 32082

## POTENTIALLY TOXIC METALS

| METALS | RESULT µg/g CREAT | REFERENCE RANGE | WITHIN REFERENCE RANGE | ELEVATED | VERY ELEVATED |
|---|---|---|---|---|---|
| Aluminum | 3.6 | < 60 | ▮ | | |
| Antimony | < dl | < 1.5 | | | |
| Arsenic | 21 | < 130 | ▬ | | |
| Beryllium | < dl | < 0.6 | | | |
| Bismuth | < dl | < 20 | | | |
| Cadmium | 0.3 | < 2 | ▬ | | |
| Lead | 0.6 | < 5 | ▬ | | |
| Mercury | 0.5 | < 5 | ▮ | | |
| Nickel | 2.1 | < 15 | ▬ | | |
| Platinum | < dl | < 1 | | | |
| Thallium | 0.3 | < 1.1 | ▬ | | |
| Thorium | < dl | < 0.5 | | | |
| Tin | < dl | < 15 | | | |
| Tungsten | 0.2 | < 1.5 | ▬ | | |
| Uranium | < dl | < 0.2 | | | |

## CREATININE

| | RESULT mg/dL | REFERENCE RANGE | 2SD LOW | 1SD LOW | MEAN | 1SD HIGH | 2SD HIGH |
|---|---|---|---|---|---|---|---|
| Creatinine | 170 | 25 - 180 | | | | ▬▬▬ | |

## SPECIMEN DATA

Comments:
| | | | | |
|---|---|---|---|---|
| Date Collected: | 1/22/2008 | Method: ICP-MS | Collection Period: | timed: 6 hours |
| Date Received: | 1/24/2008 | <dl: less than detection limit | Volume: | |
| Date Completed: | 1/30/2008 | Provoking Agent: | Provocation: | POST PROVOCATIVE |

Toxic metals are reported as µg/g creatinine to account for urine dilution variations. **Reference ranges are representative of a healthy population under non-challenge or non-provoked conditions.** No safe reference levels for toxic metals have been established.

V10.00

©DOCTOR'S DATA, INC. • ADDRESS: 3755 Illinois Avenue, St. Charles, IL 60174-2420 • CLIA ID NO: 14D0646470 • MEDICARE PROVIDER NO: 148453

# Chapter XV

# Methylation

*No, it's not Meth.*
*Meth is unhealthy.*
*This is a book on how to get healthy.*
*And my story of biomedical interventions.*
*And life.*
*And philosophy.*
*And the end of the world.*
*Which is not 2012.*
*Or is it?*

If by now you haven't figured out how complex your body is, you obviously have been sleeping through the book while looking intelligent at the same time (tricky you). If you have been dozing off, before tossing my book into the fire, make sure you buy 10 copies to create a giant explosion.

Anyway, there is a lot going on in your body on a cellular level to keep things happening. Here is a map of some of the biochemical processes taking place:

Next Page ⇨

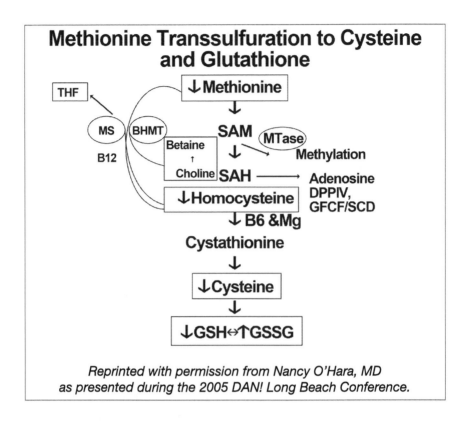

**Methionine Transsulfuration to Cysteine and Glutathione**

THF

↓Methionine

MS  BHMT

B12

SAM  MTase

Betaine ↑

Methylation

Choline SAH ────→ Adenosine

↓Homocysteine

DPPIV, GFCF/SCD

↓ B6 &Mg

Cystathionine

↓

↓Cysteine

↓

↓GSH⟷↑GSSG

*Reprinted with permission from Nancy O'Hara, MD*
*as presented during the 2005 DAN! Long Beach Conference.*

Whew! That is complicated!

Two very important biochemical pathways that keep you feeling good are called Methylation and Sulfation. Methylation and Sulfation:

- Keep DNA working properly
- Help neurotransmitters work
- Reduce inflammation
- Assist in detoxification
- Produce GLUTATHIONE (pronounced glue-ta-thigh-on.)

When I heard the word glutathione, the first thing that came to mind was "Gluten." Gluten, I believed, was bad. Recently I figured out that glutathione was not related to gluten and was not bad. Indeed, glutathione is your body's best cleaner-upper, not unlike a janitor who cleans up a building full of lawyers who have puked all over the place. If you don't have enough Glutathione, you will be a mess. Period. Glutathione cleans up toxins in your body and carries them away.

Even if you have bad genes in this area (THAT IS NOT YOUR FAULT, if you must know), doing things I've written about in this book – diet, supplementation, detoxification - may significantly help. Of particular use are MB12 shots – a star performer for improving Methylation. Also, some people need B6 and Folate.

Problems with Methylation and Sulfation are often involved in brain problems like ADHD, autism and depression. If you are having problems in these areas, work with a DAN! doctor to get it sorted out.

# Chapter XVI

# HBOT

Do you recall when I wrote that my brother and I went to California for brain SPECT scans? And, that the scans had revealed that some parts of my brain had too much activity while other parts had too little? The underactive parts of my brain were not getting enough oxygen. Naturally, that is problematic. Fortunately, there is an intervention to help with this situation: H-BOT. HBOT stands for Hyperbaric Oxygen Treatment.

If you've seen Top Gun, Independence Day, or any other movie that is nothing like the Air Force but makes you want to join, you know that the pilots in combat wear air masks over their faces. This is because when they are at higher elevations, they have a hard time taking in the air. On ground level it can also be used effectively to supercharge your oxygenation too.

In HBOT, you are placed in an airtight chamber with an oxygen mask. Gradually the internal air pressure is increased to a level around 1.3-1.5 atmospheres. The pressure experienced by the user is similar to the pressure experienced by a passenger in an airplane take off. Once desired internal pressure is achieved, rather then your head exploding, you should adjust fairly quickly.

For those who want to know, HBOT is not magic. Physics can explain the principles behind this practice. (Is this book making all your science classes come to life?) One law of physics states that when a gas is under pressure, it is likely to dissolve into a liquid. In

HBOT, that gas is oxygen and under pressure it dissolves into the liquid plasma of your blood. Once inside your circulatory system this oxygen rich blood will go to your oxygen-deficient areas.

There are two types of HBOT chambers. The first one is a Hard Chamber.

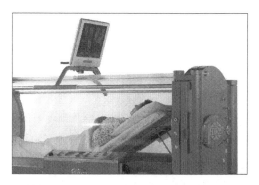

*http://emedicine.medscape.com/article/1464149-overview*

These are offered in specialized facilities. The hard chamber that I used was similar to a cockpit in a plane. There was a comfortable seat inside the chamber and I could also look through the glass in the "Cockpit" and watch a movie with subtitles. (Unfortunately, I couldn't get any audio.) As the name suggests, the sides of the chamber were hard.

Alternatively there are Soft Chambers.

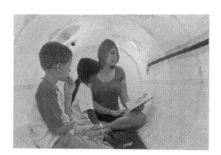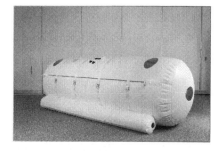

*http://en.wikipedia.org/wiki/Hyperbaric_medicine*

Seriously, these look like giant cylinder shaped bags. Most of the time you have to lie down on a mattress placed for you at the bottom. Like the hard chamber, I was given an air mask. The sides of this chamber were soft.

Most people believe that hard chambers are superior to soft chambers. There are a couple major advantages to hard chambers. To begin with, hard Chambers offer 100% pure oxygen. This is obviously the highest oxygen content available. Soft chambers are generally used with oxygen concentrators which take oxygen from the room and well...... concentrate it. The oxygen delivered to the user is much higher than the oxygen available in the room air, but much lower than the oxygen available through hard chambers.

Additionally, hard chambers offer 1.5 atmospheres of pressure or more, while soft chambers offer only around 1.3 atmospheres of pressure. However, unless your goal is to make your head explode, 1.5 is a good number.

There are some big advantages of soft chambers, though. First, they are massively convenient. They can be rented and placed in your house. Being able to complete HBOT sessions in your own home is mighty convenient. It tends to make life easier. Also, it means there's no long drive every Tuesday and Thursday (or whatever days you have it). The second advantage is cost. It is far, far cheaper.

Of course, you have to be sure that this is for you. Ask a qualified doctor if this is ok. (This book is basically entirely telling you "Go talk to your doctor.") People who have a history of seizures should

BE CAREFUL! It takes about 15 minutes to decompress, and if you exit the chamber without decompressing, you can be in big trouble.

I have sat through a total of 10 hard chamber sessions and 100 soft chamber sessions. (As I said, soft chambers are much more accessible.) After each session I found I could breathe easier and stronger while exercising. My energy level was good (which was a shocker), and it was a very calming experience to be inside a chamber. If you can do it, I recommend doing it very highly.

# Chapter XVII

# Other Interventions We Have Tried
### (Or rather, ones that have been forced upon me)

In addition to following the DAN! protocol for the past 3 years, my mom also investigated other complementary interventions. Recently mom's friend suggested Advanced Allergy Therapeutics – www.allergytx.com. This treatment retrains the immune system so it won't respond negatively to things that aren't harmful. The system can test for hundreds of potential allergens in 4 categories: contactant (touched stuff), inhalant (stuff you breath), ingestant (things you eat) or injectant (stuff shot into you with needles.) Then one by one (and appointment by appointment) the allergy symptoms are eliminated.

I realize this intervention sounds a little "out there," but it actually works! No needles, no lab tests, no pills, and no reason not to try it other than expense. The practitioner identified that my brother was allergic to his own digestive enzymes and neurotransmitters. After treatment any remaining "tummy trouble" my brother had was gone and he thought more clearly. I was allergic to several foods and some supplements. After the treatment I too felt better.

Another alternative intervention we tried was Interactive Metronome (IM) – www.interactivemetronome.com. We tried this 2 years into the DAN! protocol. IM basically works on your ability to do a sequence of tasks while keeping rhythm. It's much harder then it sounds… it's always timed to the millisecond. It has been clinically shown to help:

- Auditory competence
- Visual competence
- Tactility and Proprioception
- Gross Motor and Mobility
- Fine Motor and Manual competence
- Vestibular function and Coordination
- Language and Communication
- Long and Short Term Memory
- Auditory sequential processing
- Auditory tonal processing
- Visual sequential processing
- Central nervous system organization
- Academic performance

For my brother IM helped him keep a beat while singing and clapping. My mom also thought it helped him with math and spelling. IM was pretty easy for me, so we stopped after only a dozen sessions.

Then there was the neurodevelopmental program. This is like a "do it yourself" home based Occupational Therapy (OT), Physical Therapy (PT) and Speech program to help individuals "self-actualize." After an initial evaluation by a neurodevelopementalist, a program participant is given a customized program to do under the direction of their parents.

Your brain can be improved with the practice and stimulation this program provides, however, it's a lot of work. Tons of work. **TONS of work**. Big time investment here, don't bother with it if you aren't able to commit the time.

My mom used it with my brother with very good success. While the DAN! protocol helped my brother restore his health, this intervention helped to remediate some of the milestones he missed during development. For example, the practitioner identified that my brother was actually left handed – even though he was functioning as a right handed individual. This made sense to my mom because we have a lot of left handed individuals in both sides of my family. Mom remembered that David had a hard time deciding whether he was left or right handed when he was 5 years old. So, she guided him to the right side – thinking life would be easier for him as a right handed person. At the age of 10, David had to change his hand and eye dominance to the left side as a result of his neurodevelopmental evaluation. This took a lot of work, but mom was pleased with the results in the end. He functioned at a higher academic level and his hand writing actually improved.

For more information on this type of program you can visit:

- National Association for Child Development – www.nacd.org
- Institute for the Development of Human Potential
  – www.iahp.org
- Hope and a Future – www.hope-future.org

Finally, there was EEG biofeedback training, which we used prior to working with a DAN! doctor. This one was fairly simple... just have the doctor put a couple wires on your head and then you play a computer game. Rather then use an Xbox 360 controller, you control the game with your mind. Before you ask, this isn't as cool as it may sound. In some games you may play, your character walks forward if your brain works right, and your character stands still if your brain is not functioning optimally. Overall it's good for your brain and I had fun, but my mom thinks we would have gotten better results if we tried it after working with Dr. Kartzinel for a while.

# Chapter XVIII

# Conclusion

I'm coming up to the end of this epic adventure, as far as the book goes. To sum it up, I had an unhealthy body that made my brain appear broken. I had trouble sustaining attention and maintaining energy. Mom thought I lacked interest in life. Additionally, I was plagued by acid reflux. While all my teachers thought I was very bright, in 2nd grade I had a tested IQ of 101 – painfully average. The tester told my mom my attention span impacted the results. Clearly, I had issues.

After 3 years on the DAN! protocol, coupled with other interventions, I am doing much better. My acid reflux is gone and I feel strong and energetic. I love to exercise and do sports! Sustaining attention is no longer an issue for me either. In fact, recently I took a standardized test called the Woodcock-Johnson Test of Achievement (sounds very professional, don't you think?). Although I'm in the 8th grade I scored at the college level in Math and English. The results indicate that my brain has been fixed!

Next Page ⇨

# H.I.S. Place
For Help in Schooling
**Judith B. Munday**
1204 Murray Drive Chesapeake VA 23322
757-482-5709   877-418-6264
learn@helpinschool.net   www.helpinschool.net

TESTING REPORT

Summary and Score Report                                                          Page 2
Zimmermann, Andrew
March 19, 2010

TABLE OF SCORES
*Woodcock-Johnson III Normative Update Tests of Achievement (Form A)*
WJ III NU Compuscore and Profiles Program, Version 3.1
Norms based on age 14-4

| CLUSTER/Test | Age Equiv | Development | RPI | SS (90% Band) | Grade Equiv |
|---|---|---|---|---|---|
| BRIEF ACHIEVEMENT | 30 | advanced | 99/90 | 119 (114-124) | 13.0 |
| BRIEF READING | 24 | advanced | 98/90 | 116 (109-122) | 13.0 |
| BRIEF MATH | >30 | v advanced | 100/90 | 128 (122-134) | >18.0 |
| BRIEF WRITING | >30 | advanced | 98/90 | 118 (111-125) | 13.6 |
| ACADEMIC SKILLS | 25 | advanced | 98/90 | 117 (111-123) | 13.0 |
| ACADEMIC APPS | >30 | advanced | 99/90 | 128 (122-133) | >18.0 |
| Letter-Word Identification | 16-2 | approp to adv | 96/90 | 108 (101-115) | 10.7 |
| Passage Comprehension | >30 | advanced | 99/90 | 121 (111-131) | >18.0 |
| Calculation | >23 | advanced | 99/90 | 122 (114-130) | >18.0 |
| Applied Problems | >30 | v advanced | 100/90 | 124 (118-130) | >18.0 |
| Spelling | 19 | approp to adv | 96/90 | 108 (101-115) | 13.0 |
| Writing Samples | >30 | advanced | 99/90 | 125 (115-135) | >18.0 |

- 82 -

David took the Woodcock-Johnson in 5th grade and scored at grade level. In 6th grade he took the test again and his test results went up 3 grade levels thanks to all the interventions discussed in this book.

**H.I.S. Place**
For Help in Schooling
**Judith B. Munday**
1204 Murray Drive Chesapeake VA 23322
757-482-5709   877-418-6264
learn@helpinschool.net   www.helpinschool.net

TESTING REPORT

Summary and Score Report                                                          Page 2
Zimmermann, David
March 15, 2010

TABLE OF SCORES
*Woodcock-Johnson III Normative Update Tests of Achievement (Form A)*
WJ III NU Compuscore and Profiles Program, Version 3.1
Norms based on age 12-1

| CLUSTER/Test | Age Equiv | Development | RPI** | SS (90% Band) | Grade Equiv |
|---|---|---|---|---|---|
| BRIEF ACHIEVEMENT | 14-11 | approp to adv | 97/90 | 115 (109-120) | 9.4 |
| ORAL EXPRESSION | 12-11 | age-approp | 92/90 | 103 (96-111) | 7.5 |
| BROAD READING | 13-7 | approp to adv | 95/90 | 109 (103-115) | 8.2 |
| BROAD MATH | 15-7 | approp to adv | 97/90 | 116 (110-121) | 10.2 |
| BRIEF READING | 13-5 | age-approp | 95/90 | 107 (100-114) | 8.0 |
| BRIEF MATH | 15-8 | approp to adv | 98/90 | 115 (108-121) | 10.2 |
| MATH CALC SKILLS | 15-11 | approp to adv | 97/90 | 117 (110-124) | 10.6 |
| BRIEF WRITING | 27 | advanced | 98/90 | 124 (116-131) | 13.0 |
| ACADEMIC SKILLS | 15-0 | advanced | 98/90 | 117 (111-123) | 9.6 |
| ACADEMIC APPS | 16-3 | approp to adv | 97/90 | 113 (108-119) | 10.8 |
| Letter-Word Identification | 12-11 | age-approp | 94/90 | 105 (98-111) | 7.5 |
| Reading Fluency | 14-0 | approp to adv | 96/90 | 108 (103-114) | 8.6 |
| Passage Comprehension | 14-8 | approp to adv | 95/90 | 108 (98-118) | 9.2 |
| Calculation | 16-6 | advanced | 98/90 | 116 (106-125) | 11.0 |
| Math Fluency | 1 15-6 | approp to adv | 96/90 | 114 (110-119) | 10.0 |
| Applied Problems | 15-4 | approp to adv | 97/90 | 109 (103-115) | 9.8 |
| Spelling | 23 | advanced | 99/90 | 119 (112-127) | 13.0 |
| Writing Samples | >30 | advanced | 98/90 | 118 (108-129) | 13.0 |
| Story Recall | >20 | approp to adv | 97/90 | 135 (121-148) | >13.3 |
| Story Recall-Delayed | >29 | age-approp | 94/90 | 116 (104-128) | >17.8 |

If your brain is broken, do what I did. Assess the situation first. Look over what's been happening. If you believe in God, Allah, Zeus, or some other deity, pray about it. If you aren't religious, I'm not going to say pray about it but rather do some self-reflection. After that, find a good DAN! doctor. Or, if you can't find a DAN! doctor look for good doctor who specializes in integrative medicine or functional medicine. Even a naturopath who has experience in ASD and ADHD might help. You don't have to try as many interventions as I did, but once you start experiencing success you might start getting addicted to it!

The brain is a very amazing organ. All of our lives are possible because of 3 pounds of grey matter. You can change your brain. Anyone can. All you need is excellent medical advice, some extra cash, and a will to succeed. All of the sacrifices I made were worth the pain. I am now quite productive and feel awesome! Thank you, God! And thanks mom, too!

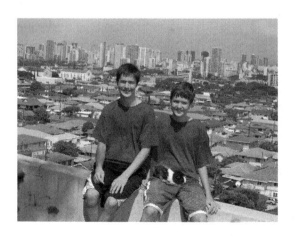

# Bonus Section

Now for my weight loss/health optimization plan. It's a fairly simple one. I split it up into 3 parts: Diet, Exercise, and Final Thoughts.

First, there is the diet. This is a real easy one. For you fellow dudes, it means you have to choose between "Burger King" and "Ladies King." For the women, choose between "Dairy Queen" and "Prom Queen" or something. If you chose the former, please stop reading this section, it won't help you.

To start off, you'll likely want to pick up the diet I did – gluten free/casein free (GF/CF). This means no dairy, no gluten, and no soy. Fairly easy concept to understand, very difficult to pull off. I won't sugarcoat this for you... it's not easy. If you isolate yourself from society and simply feast off whole foods, it's pretty easy. Most people want to engage with society on this planet, however. So here are a couple things you need to do when you get invited to a party and don't want to seem like a freak.

a) *Fake it.* Bring your own diet approved food to the table. When someone says "Dude! Have some of the pizza, it's great!" usually you want to respond with "I would... but I've had so many pretzels (the gluten free ones you brought, tricky you), I can't eat any more." If they see you eating later, simply say, "I was hungry again." Either way, you win.

b) *Tell the host of your dietary limitations, assuming the host is not a creep.* There's a good chance the host will try to accommodate you, assuming you trust the host not to tell the world. If you don't, why are you going? Are you attempting to crash the party and ruin it for everyone else? The host should make sure that there's something that can be set aside, or at least find out what's approved.

c) *Take your mind off the bloody food.* Life does not revolve around eating. True, it is tormenting to avoid foods at a party, but this diet takes some willpower. Losing weight, for that matter takes willpower. If you can't bring up some willpower and some commitment, the first step, for me anyway, is to find a sport.

Assuming you like it, I find martial arts are a great way to grow willpower. (I also think it is important for everyone, male and female, to take some kind of martial arts class. Women, if all they have is grappling, you are excused.) Wrestling also works well. Jogging is terrific. My mom makes David and I jog 2 miles every day as part of our homeschool requirements. While I don't always like to start a jog, when I return I feel alert and fantastic. Some researchers believe that jogging actually increases your brain cells.

But what DOES NOT work well is golf and bowling, or some other non-physical sport.

If you are in your 60s and actually reading my book (Yippy!), life has probably helped you develop strong willpower. If not, time to pick up the running shoes and go. (But if you are 60+ you might want to get a doctor's clearance and a stationary bicycle!)

My personal workout routine is Brazilian Jijitsu (my favorite martial art), wrestling, track, midsection workouts, weights, sometimes swimming, and taking a ride on the standup paddle with my dad.

Before you ask, by "Take a ride" I push myself on my own board. Here's my dad:

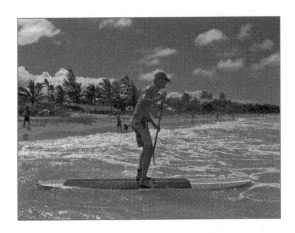

In the end though, if you get a workout and you like it, go straight ahead and pursue any exercise you wish. If you hate it, but it makes you healthier than Brian Clay, I'd look for something else. If you don't have a passion for the sport you are pursuing, it will be a real drag to practice, and you'll end up leaving.

Similarly, say I was going to join a gym. What should I join, a gym that's close and decent that I'll hit 3 times a week or an award-winning gym much further away that I'll probably only visit 3 times a year? Let's say your gym membership is… for easy math $450 a year. If you only visit 3 times a year your cost per visit is $150.00! Also, if you hit the gym 3 times a year, each time is going to be quite painful, and you aren't going to get much out of the session. Go with the less glamorous gym that is convenient.

One more note….an exercise you definitely need to do - *Midsection workouts*. My philosophy is because no two objects may occupy the same space at the same time, popping in several dozen crunches, leg raises, sit-ups, knee-ups, and side sit-ups will get you closer to the 6-pack abs you've dreamed of while conquering a bulging mid-section. Once you get the abs, away goes the fatness. I've held this philosophy for a long time, and then David Zinczenko turned it into a book.

Now reading about a diet and exercise program is much easier than implementing one. Here are my final thoughts and 10 commandments for health and fitness:

1. *Thou shalt not get jacked up on booze, cigarettes, or drugs.*
2. *Thou shalt not eat wheat or dairy until approved by your DAN! doctor.*
3. *Thou shalt exercise restraint.*
4. *Thou shalt not restrain to exercise.*
5. *If it be thy wish, thou may eat at a fast-food restaurant off-season once every other week at absolute maximum. On-season, fast-food is out.*
6. *Thou shalt reward thineself, but not with fast food. I watch fights online.*
7. *Thou shalt speak to thy doctor about a fitness plans.*
8. *Thou shalt listen to thy doctor.*
.9 *Thou shalt push thineself.*
10. *Thou shalt check nutrition facts.*
11. *And most importantly of all: Thou shalt not quit when thee has shrunk several sizes.*
12. *Finally, thou shalt not care about losing count of commandments.*

This may not be an easy project for you. It isn't easy for anyone (except maybe experienced bodybuilders). But as Dwayne Johnson would say, "Hard work ALWAYS pays off." Push yourself beyond what you think you can do, because you'll likely end up doing less than you can do. There's also the matter of overtraining but not many people have to worry about that.

As I've said far too many times in this book (and I will say it again), if you don't pay attention to your body, when you need to use your body it won't pay attention to you. After all, why should it?

*********************************************************************************

Want to talk with me and other kids undergoing biomedical interventions? Join us on Facebook at Biomed Kids.

Made in the USA
Columbia, SC
07 June 2019